Natural Remedies:

Amazing Organic Scrubs Recipes for Your Face and Body with Herbs and Essential Oils

Table of content:

Introduction - You need an alternative

You've looked everywhere for advice on how to make your hair and skin healthier, and you've gotten is advice on what shampoos, facial masks and scrubs to buy, but you don't want that. You want to be able to take control of your skin products.

You've looked online to find advice on natural alternatives, and you found more information than you can sift through. Look no further. This book is written to get your started in making scrubs that are both herbal and essential based. It will explain every ingredient, what each of the essential oils and herbs do, how long the scrubs last, and how to make and use them. Your starter guide to putting the power and choice of maintaining your skin and hair is all in these pages. What are you waiting for?

Chapter 1 - Natural Health 101

When I say *Natural Health*, I am referring to the practice of maintaining a healthy body, mind, and spirit, otherwise known as Holistic healing. It is the belief that all illnesses have a root cause that must be addressed from the cause and not the symptoms. Here is an example:

You feel ill. You've been feeling ill for a while. You decide to go to a Natural Health practitioner instead of a mainstream doctor. When they call you back to a room, the doctor enters and asks how you're feeling, what your symptoms are, and then he also asks if the symptoms are worse during the day, afternoon, or evening. He asks about your work schedule, your hobbies, your diet, and other things a mainstream doctor would not normally ask. This is because the Naturopath is trying to get to know you and not your illness. He may recommend changes in routine and diet, may list remedies to take and how often to take them. This is because he is treating you and not the illness. You see, by making changes to your diet, giving you ways to cope with stress, and also suggesting ways to change your routine, he is helping treat the root cause of the illness, and the rest will handle itself.

Natural health has been practiced for millennia and the first real documentation of such natural health practices started in China. This practice was handed down from practitioner to apprentice and is known today as *Traditional Chinese Medicine*. Other countries have there forms as well. India has Ayurveda. France was the birthplace of Aromatherapy. All very potent practices which have become pushed aside by mainstream medicine and practices. It started making a come-back in the mid to early nineties, but most people labeled it "new age". Today, you can find Homeopaths, Naturopaths ,and practitioners of Aromatherapy online and locally.

Aloe *(Aloe Vera)*

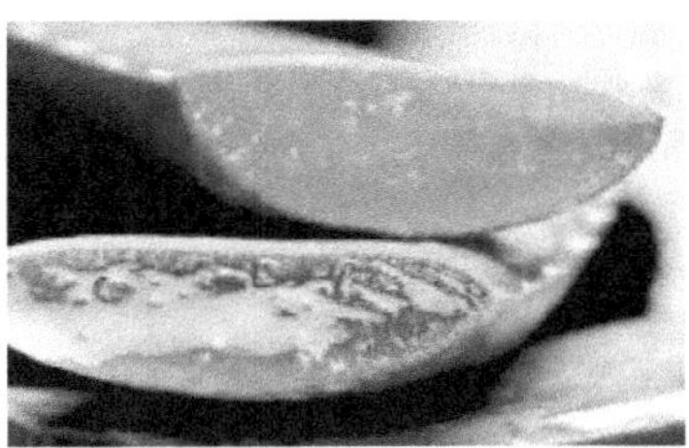

This is a well known herb for skin problems. It can be used for scrubs, using the juice as the carrier for the essential oils.

Bilberry *(Vaccinium myrtullus)*

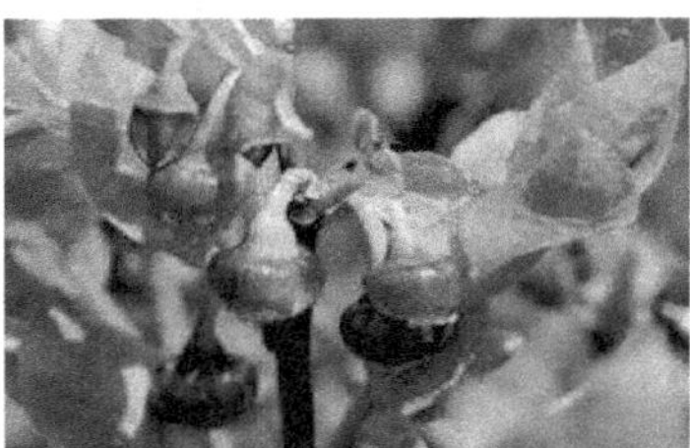

This herb has antibacterial properties that can help speed healing for rashes, fungus, and scrapes.

Calendula (Marigold) *(Calendula officinalis)*

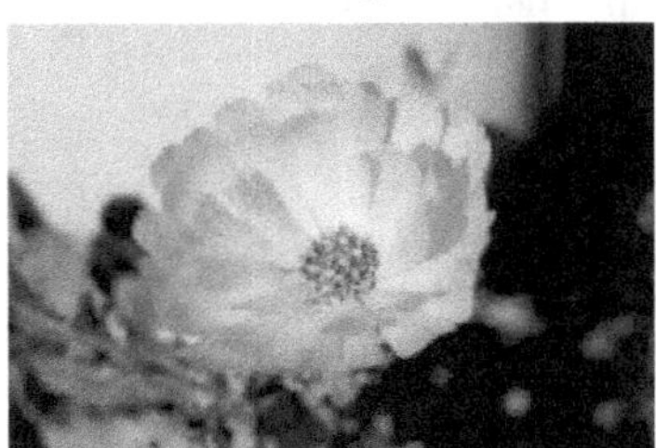

These flower petals have been used to treat bruises, helps the heal cuts and scraps, and can also help treat other skin problems as well.

Chamomile, Roman (*Anthemis nobilis*)

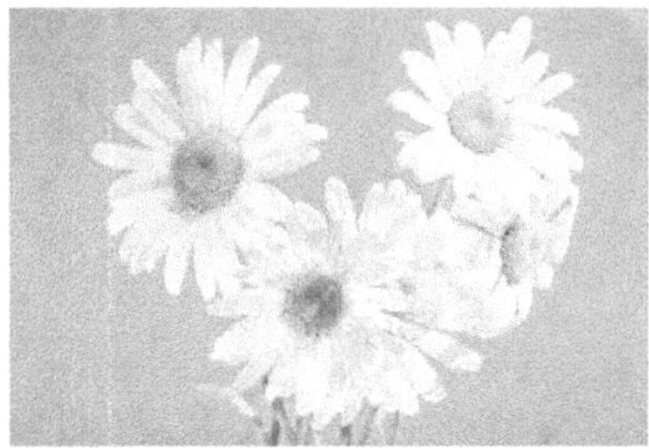

This is a perfect herbal for smoothing out and healing skin abrasions, rashes, and preventing acne.

Comfrey (*Symphytum officinale*)

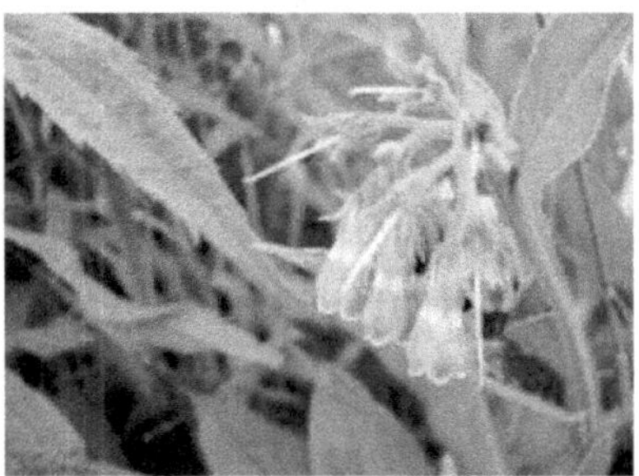

This herb is often used to bring boils to a head in order to drain them. It is also effective in treating burns and swelling.

Gotu Kola *(Hydrocotyle asiatica)*

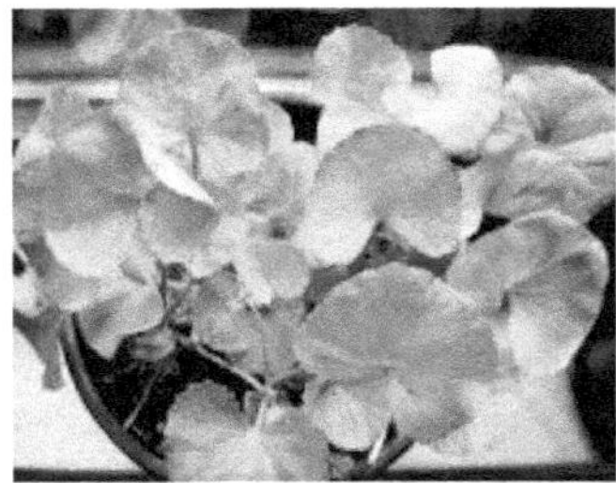

This is used on occasion to help treat psoriasis.

Peppermint *(Mentha piperita)*

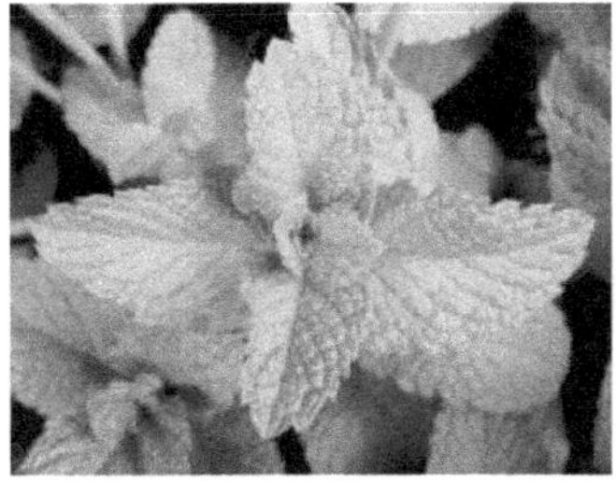

This herb is good to add into scrubs to get rid of bacteria and help remove infections. It also stimulates the skin.

St. John's Wort *(Hypericum perforatum)*

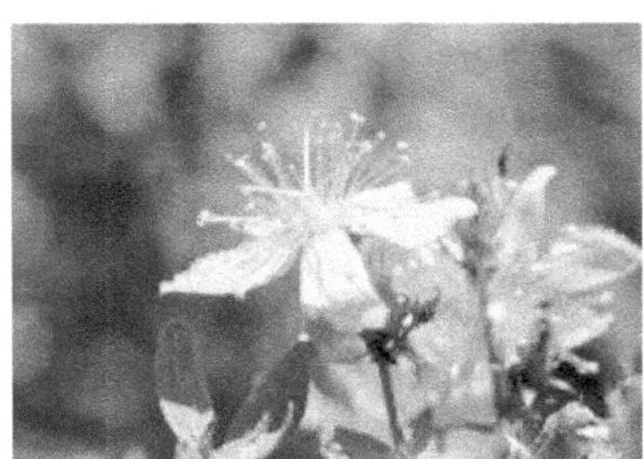

This is an herb used in the scrubs to help with skin problems and as a first aid treatment for bug bites. Do not use this herb if you are taking anti-depressants as this herb can boost the actions of those types of medications.

Tumeric *(Curcuma longa)*

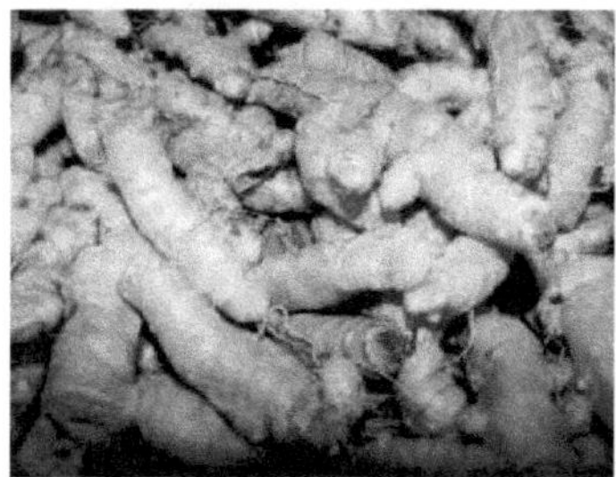

This herb's antibacterial and anti-fungal properties can help to treat athlete's foot and other fungal problems.

Carrot Seed *(Daucus carota)*

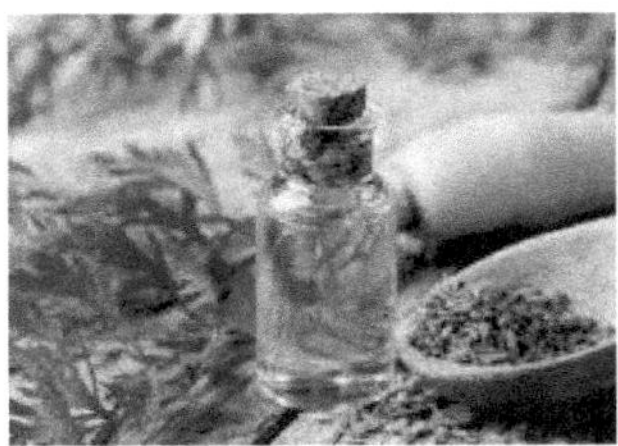

This oil is used in small doses, but is quite effective in treating dermatitis, eczema, psoriasis, and can also make the skin healthier.

Frankincense *(Boswellia carteri)*

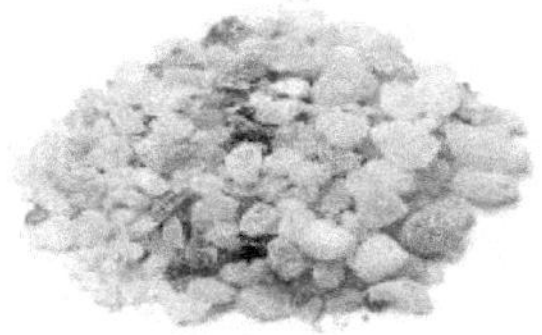

Making scrubs with this essential oil can help with blemishes, more mature complexions, scars, wrinkles, and dry skin.

Geranium *(Pelargonium graveolens)*

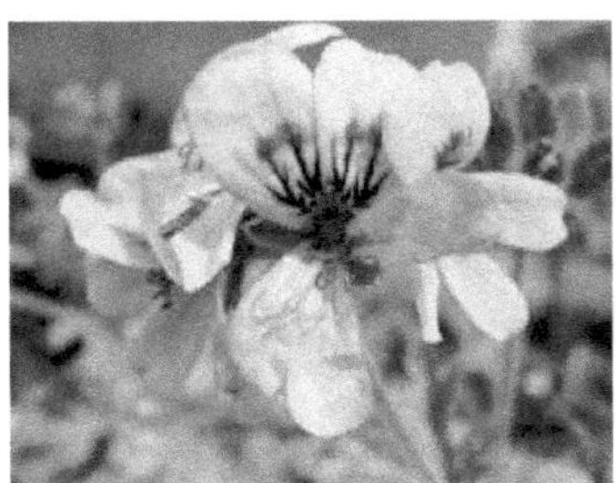

This oil helps with broken capillaries, clogged pores, and other skin conditions.

Lavender *(Lavandula angustifolia)*

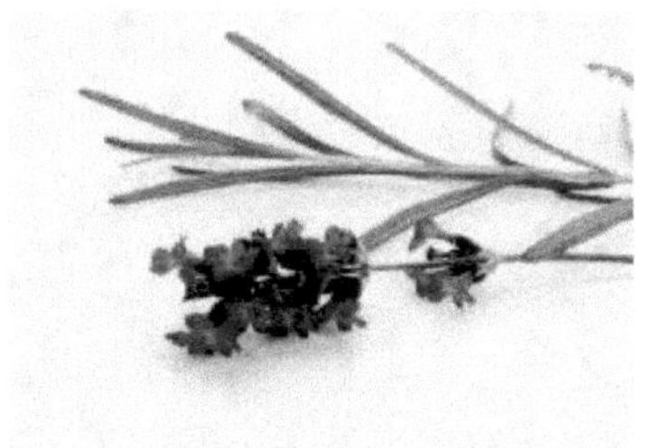

This is an essential oil that comes highly recommended when it comes to treating burns, abrasions, rashes, and other skin problems.

Myrrh *(Commiphora myrrha)*

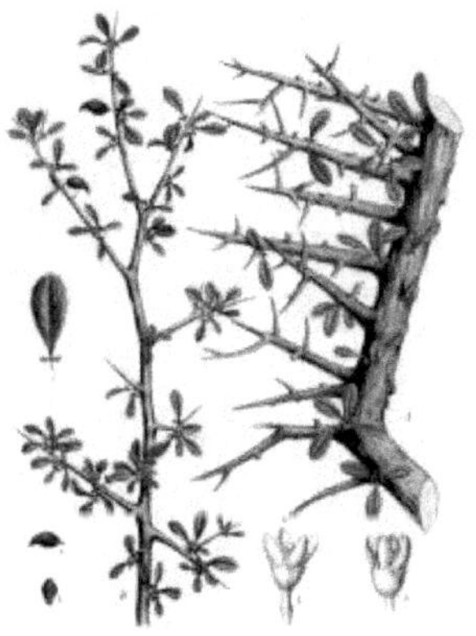

This is another essential oil that is good for more mature skin types, psoriasis and chapped skin.

Patchouli *(Pogostemon cablin)*

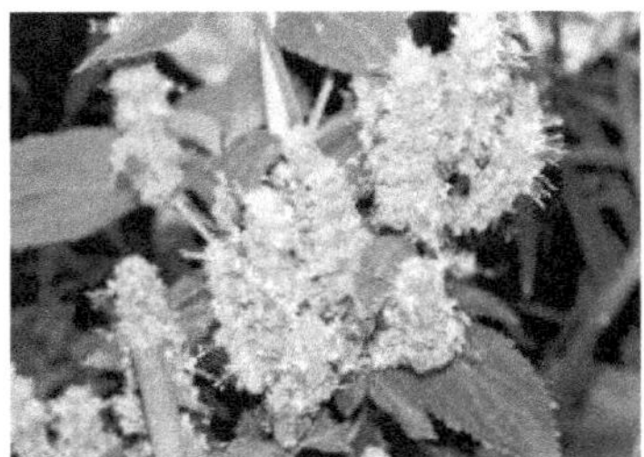

Most famous for being used in the 60's by hippies, this oil is effective in treating weeping psoriasis and eczema, acne, and fungal infections.

Rose *(Rosa x damascena)*

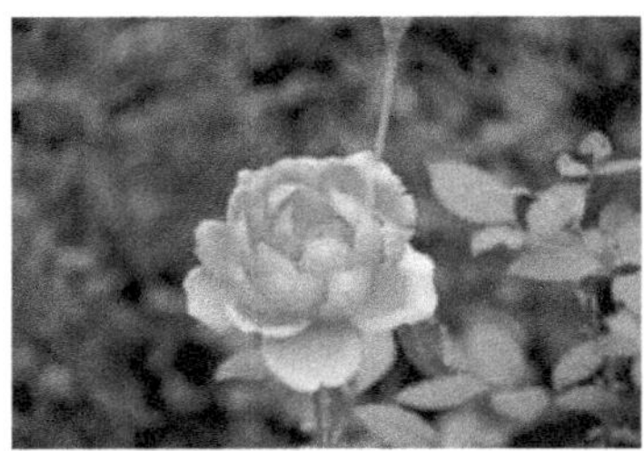

Most commonly used in blends for mature complexions, wrinkles, and dry skin conditions.

Tea Tree *(Melaleuca alternifolia)*

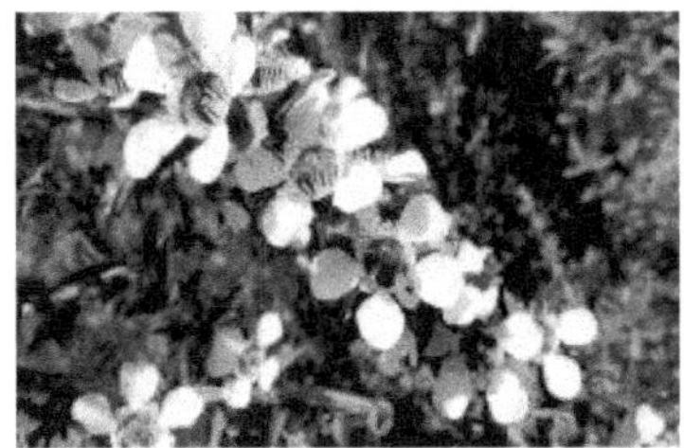

This is mainly used as a disinfectant. It is also great for treating athlete's foot, oily skin and also a treatment for dandruff.

Ylang Ylang *(Cananga adorata)*

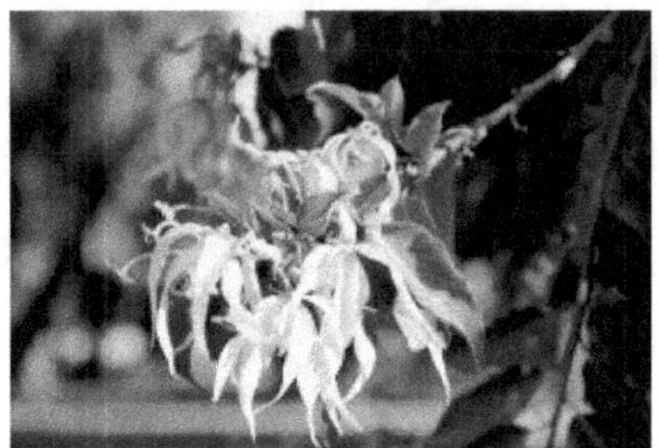

This soothes skin irritations, oily skin, and is used for general skin care.

Cedarwood, Atlas *(Cedrus atlantica)*

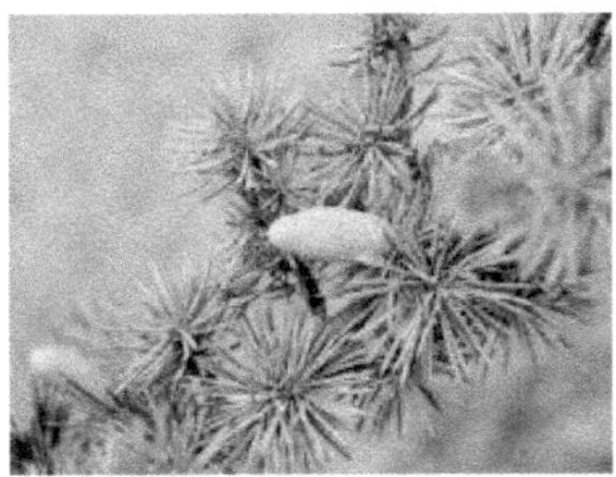

This essential oil is not only good for oily skin conditions, but it added to blends for dandruff and hair loss.

Clary Sage *(Salvia sclarea)*

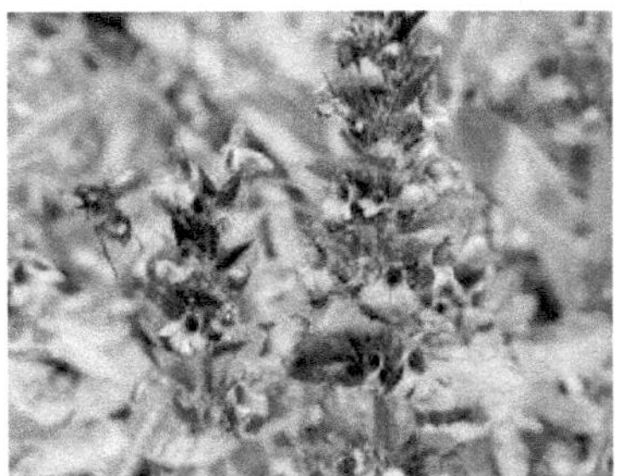

This essential oil is good for treating hair loss, dandruff, and also has been known to help balance oily skin and scalp. This oil has also been known to boost the action of narcotic prescription medications.

Petitgrain *(Citrus aurantium)*

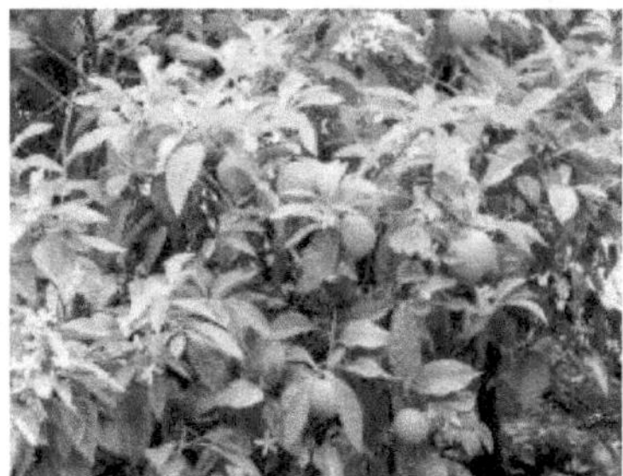

This oil helps to balance oil production in this skin and scalp.

Rosemary *(Rosmarius officinalis)*

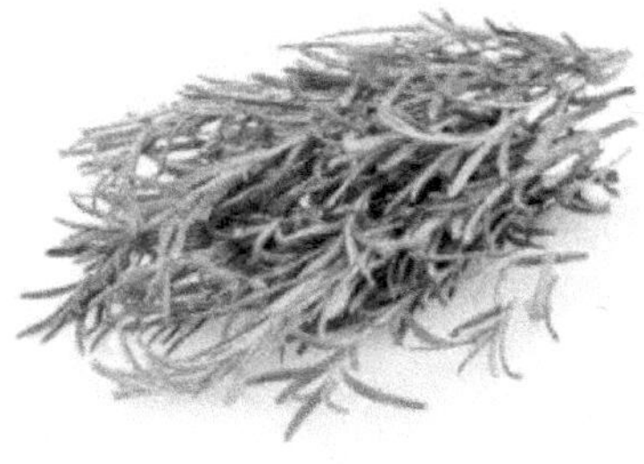

This oil helps to balance the natural oil your scalp produces, helps to promote the growing of hair, and is also good in treating dandruff and lice.

Everything needs to proper tools and making your scrubs is no different. Here is a list of things that will help you make the scrubs in this book and when you decide to try making some of your own.

Bowls

Mixing bowls that hold four cups are ideal and glass is preferred. This will let you stir the ingredients without worrying about any spilling out of the bowl. You will need two of them.

Measuring spoons and cups

These will come in handy for the sugars and salts you will be using for your scrubs.

Stirring spoons

Silicone is preferred although wooden/bamboo works well, too.

Dark colored glass jars w/ lids

This is in case you make a large batch of scrubs. The dark color of the glass will prevent sunlight from coming into the jar and evaporating the essential oils.

Labels

It's always good to label your scrubs to make sure you know which one you are wanting to use and which one you are saving for later.

Sea Salt

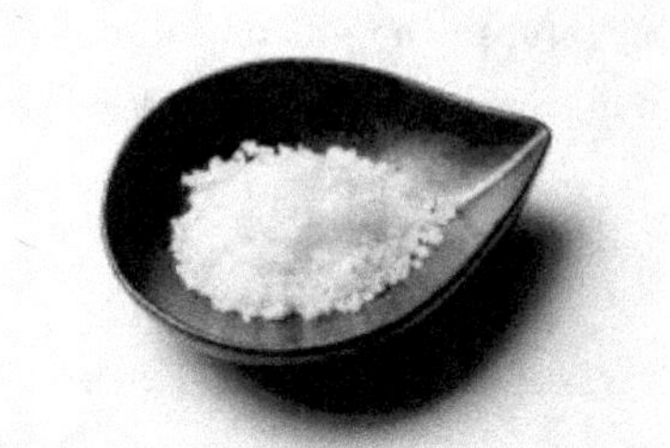

Organic is best. Salt scrubs are good for helping with overly oily skin. Small grain salt is good for regular maintenance while medium size grains are a good for exfoliating the skin for more stubborn conditions.

Sugar

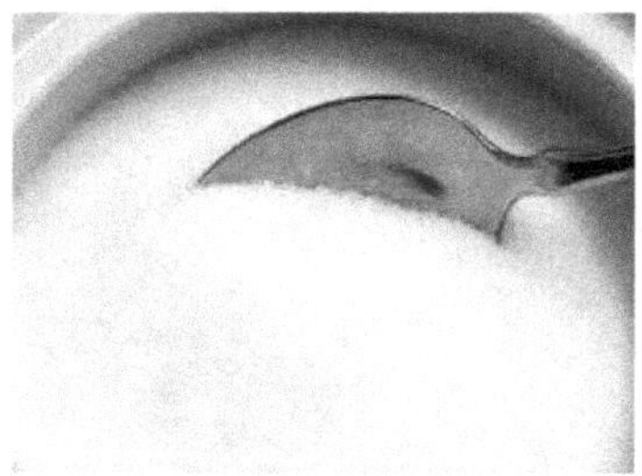

Brown sugar is often the best to use for sugar scrubs as it has the molasses usually left out during processing. The molasses has vitamins and minerals your skin needs to condition and help smooth it. If you don't have brown sugar, you can always make some by adding sulfur-free molasses to white sugar.

Rapadura is best for sugar scrubs if you can find it in course grains, but not too course. Rapadura is the sugar before it is processed.

Powdered herbs

When making scrubs, powdered herbs are the best preparation of the herbs to use. This is because they will blend easily with the sugar or salt.

Carrier oils

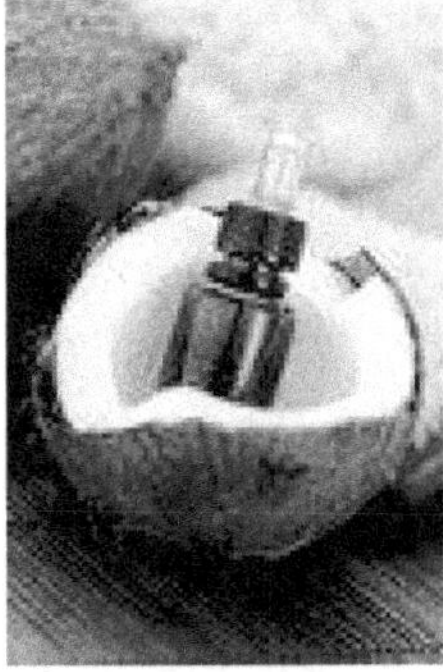

These are oils you add essential oils to in order to dilute them. The most commonly used carriers oils are Sweet Almond, Apricot Kernel, and coconut. Keep in mind, when buying the coconut oil, it will harden at room temperature unless you buy the fractionated coconut oil.

1. Always dilute your essential oils. Using them undiluted can cause dermatitis.

2. Keep essential oils and herbals out of the reach of children.

3. Shelf life of the scrubs, once they are made, is six months before the carrier oils start to break down.

4. Store the essential oils in a dark, cool place. Essential oils have a shelf life of about a year before they start lose their potency.

5. Store the powdered herbs in a cool, dry place. Powdered herbs can last up to three years, if stored in air-tight containers.

6. Do NOT apply scrubs of any kind to broken skin. This will only irritate the condition.

How to use a scrub.

1. Lightly clean the area to which you are applying the scrub.

2. Apply a thin layer of the scrub to the area and work it into the skin in circles.

3. Shower and wash it off.

4. You can use scrubs up to three times a week. You need to let your skin rest between scrubs so it can heal properly and absorb the medicinal properties of the oils and herbs.

How to make scrubs

- Mix the essential oils with the carrier oil.

- Set it aside

- Mix the sugar/salt and any dry ingredients

- Add the oils to the dry ingredients

- Place the scrub into a jar and tighten the lid.

- Let is sit overnight before using.

Chapter 2 - Facial Scrubs

Depending on your skin type, you will need different ingredients.

Oily Skin

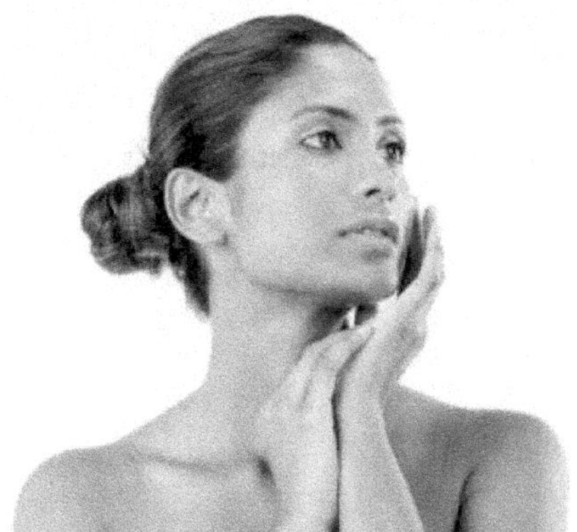

This is a skin complexion when two conditions occur:

1. Your skin produces more natural oils making your skin oily.

2. Your skin is actually dry but tries to pull moisture in from the air around it, often making the skin oily.

The best way to regulate the oils your skin produces if your complexion is due to the first problem is to track your diet and write down the foods you've eaten. There are foods you can eat that will cause your skin to produce oils.

By avoiding these foods, you can start to regulate your skin's oil production. Also, you can make sure the cleansers you're using don't dry out your skin. This could make your oily skin worse.

The second problem can be easily figured out. After cleaning your skin, time how long it takes your skin to go from dry to oily. If it takes about an hour or two before you start to see a sheen, you may have the second problem.

Try washing your face once a day and allow your face to air dry. Follow this up with a moisturizer to keep the skin soft and smooth. Washing your face more than once a day can't make your skin over into overdrive in regards to producing the natural oils your body does on its own.

Extra Ingredients for oily skin

There are things you can add to your scrub to help absorb the excess oils:

Oatmeal

Finely ground oatmeal has been known, not only to absorb excess oils, but it can also keep the skin smooth.

Clay powders

Adding a small amount of this powder to a scrub will help absorb oils from the skin.

Oily Face Scrub I

1/2 Cup brown sugar
1 tbsp Ground Peppermint
1/2 tbsp ground oatmeal
3 tbsp Sweet Almond Oil
2 Drops Clary Sage
4 Drops Petitgrain
4 Drops Ylang Ylang
2 Drops Peppermint

Oily Face Scrub II

1/2 Cup Sea Salt

1 tbsp Ground Calendula Petals

1/2 tbsp ground Clay powder

3 tbsp Sweet Almond Oil

2 Drops Altas Cedarwood

4 Drops Carrot Seed

4 Drops Tea Tree

2 Drops Myrrh

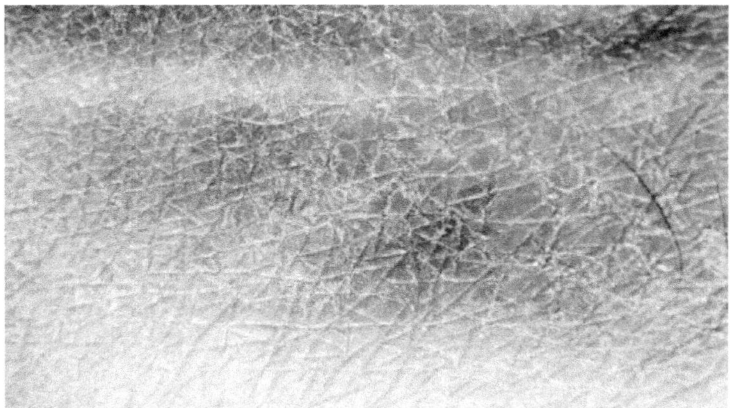

This skin type can range from a slight ashy look to eczema and psoriasis. There are a few things you can do to regulate your dry skin.

1. Moisturize your skin in the morning and before you go to bed.

2. Carry moisturizer with you in your makeup kit to apply when needed.

3. Let your skin air dry. This let's your skin soak of moisture naturally.

4. Wash with luke-warm water. Hot water will dry out your skin.

Often times eczema or psoriasis are the cause of an allergic reaction to either an environmental substance or food. Visit a specialist who can give you an allergy test to determine what food or substances could be causing the rashes.

Lack of dehydration can cause your skin to dry out, become ashy, or even start to crack. To see if you are dehydrated, pinch a small amount of skin on the top of your hand and then let go.

If the skin snaps immediately back into place, you are fine. If the skin slowly goes back to its original position, you need to hydrate. Drinking water, coconut water, or any non-alcoholic beverage, like juice, will give your body the hydration it needs to keep going.

Don't use the scrubs on cracked or broken skin.

Extra ingredients for dry skin

There are two herbs you can add to your arsenal to help you with dry skin:

Kelp

This herb is high in the vitamins and minerals your skin needs to heal and stay healthy.

Horsetail

This is another herb that can boost the action of the scrub and soften skin.

Dry Skin Scrub I

1/2 Cup Brown Sugar
1/2 tbsp Kelp
1/2 tbsp Horsetail
1 tbsp Sweet Almond oil
1 tbsp Coconut oil
6 Drops Lavender
4 Drops Patchouli
2 Drops Geranium

Dry Facial Scrub II

1/4 Cup Brown Sugar
1/4 Cup Sea Salt
1 tbsp Kelp
2 tbsp coconut oil
4 Drops Ylang Ylang
4 Drops Rose
2 Drops Frankincense
2 Drops Carrot Seed

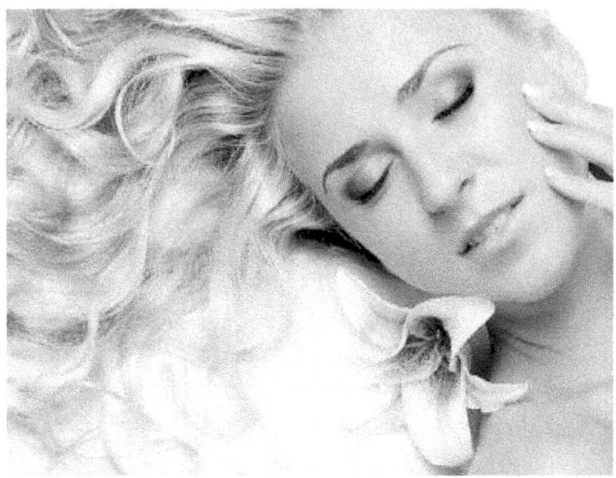

Yes, normal skin needs love and attention, too, and we haven't forgotten it.

If you have a daily regimen that works for you, keep it up. A regular routine might look like this:

-Wash face in the morning

- Moisturize after washing

-Facial mask three times a week.

-Nightly moisturizing

-Light washing after make-up removal

Regular Maintenance I

1/2 Cup Brown Sugar

3 tbsp Sweet Almond Oil

4 Drops Ylang Ylang

4 Drops Lavender

4 Drops Peppermint

3 Drops Carrot Seed

3 Drops Chamomile

Regular Maintenance II

1/2 Cup Brown Sugar
3 tbsp Sweet Almond Oil
4 Drops Chamomile
4 Drops Rose
4 Drops Ylang Ylang
3 Drops Geranium
3 Drops Lavender

Chapter 3 - Your Body

From your head to your feet, your body deserves to be pampered and cared for as much as you care for your face. You can develop rough patches on elbows and knees, your back can develop acne and dry skin patches as well. Your entire body could use scrubs for exfoliation, healing, and keeping your skin healthy.

Taking care of your body

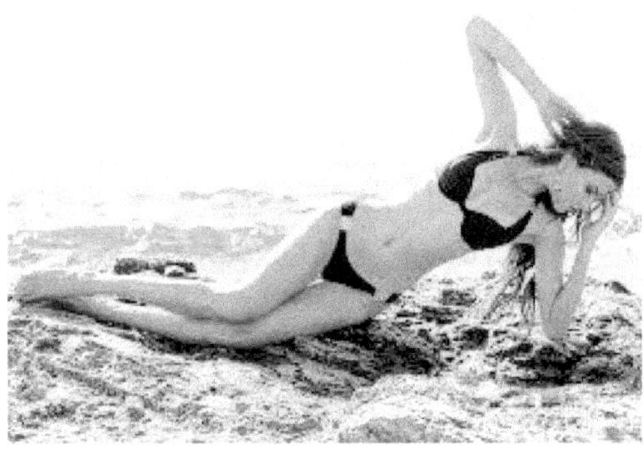

To maintain healthy skin, you have to dress for the season. If the sun is glaring at you, use sun screen or sun block. Wear hats for shade and to help prevent having a sun burn on your face.

In the winter, cover any skin to keep it from getting wind burned or frostbite. Both can leave your skin damaged.

Using a regular moisturizer can keep your skin from getting dry and damaged. Washing with luke-warm water will also help keep it from drying out. When you can, let your body air dry.

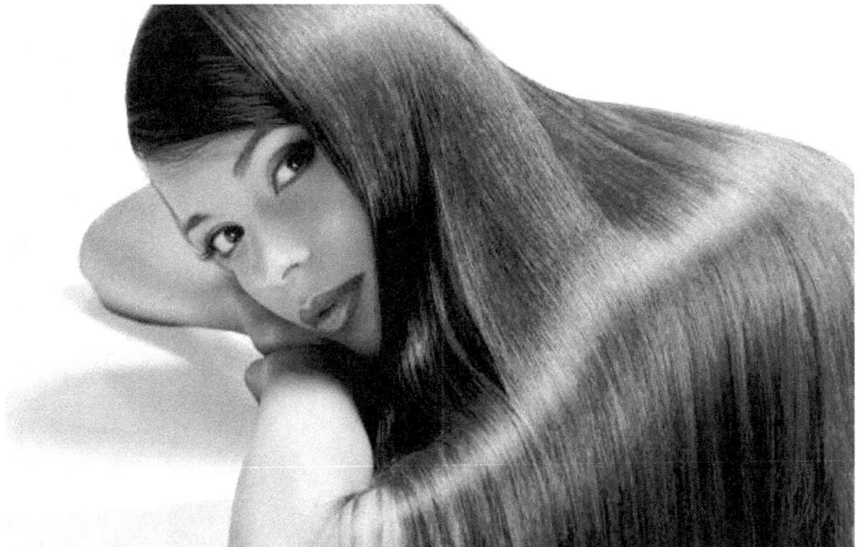

You wash it. You dry it. You style it. You add products to it to make it stay in place once you have that look you were looking for, and all of this can damage your hair leaving it dull, dry, and with split ends. The products you use can also add to build up on your scalp which can make your hair look limp.

Try This:

Put a tablespoon of conditioner in a cup and add half a cup of water. Don't stir it. Just time how long it takes for the conditioner to dissolve. It's taking a while isn't it? Just think how much of it is left on your scalp and never really washes out.

Here are a few scrubs you can use to remove the build-up, balance your scalps sebum production, and even promote hair growth.

Now, think about the residue you leave on your scalp if you use a leave-in conditioner. The build-up can get worse when you add gel, mousse, and even hair spray.

Oily Scalp

2 tbsp Brown Sugar

2 tbsp Lemon Juice

2 tbsp coconut oil

6 Drops Petitgrain

3 Drops Lavender

2 Drops Clary Sage

Dry Scalp

2 tbsp Brown Sugar

2 tbsp Lemon Juice

2 tbsp coconut oil

6 Drops Lavender

3 Drops Ylang Ylang

3 Drops Rose

Normal Scalp

2 tbsp Brown Sugar

2 tbsp Lemon Juice

2 tbsp coconut oil

6 Drops Petitgrain

Rinsing the Scrub

Now you have the oils in the your hair. You need to break them up before you continue washing your hair.

2 tbsp Apple Cider Vinegar

2 Cups Filtered Water

- Mix together
- Tilt head back
- Slowly pour it from the front of the brow and let the rinse flow backwards breaking up the oils.
- Repeat only if needed.
- Continue with the rest of the hair washing routine.

Oily back

1/4 cup Sea Salt

1/4 Cup Brown sugar

3 tbsp Coconut oil

6 Drops Tea Tree oil

3 Drops Peppermint

3 Drops Petitgrain

3 Drops Cedarwood

Dry back

1/2 Cup Brown sugar

3 tbsp Coconut oil

6 Drops of Lavender

3 Drops Patchouli

3 Drops Myrrh

3 Drops Geranium

Normal Back

1/2 Cup Brown sugar

3 tbsp Sweet Almond oil

6 Drops of Ylang Ylang

3 Drops of Neroli

3 Drops of Myrrh

Your chest

I am not talking about breasts. I am talking about the area above and below the breasts. You can use the scrubs for your breasts, but avoid the nipple area if you do. There are a couple of things you can add here as well.

Eucalyptus *(Eucalyptus globulus)*

Not only does the essential oil help with burns and and insect bites, but you can use it in a blended chest scrub to make breathing easier, too.

Oily Chest I

1/2 cup of Sea salt

3 tbsp of Sweet Almond Oil

6 Drops of Eucalyptus

3 Drops of Peppermint

Oily Chest II

1/2 cup of Sea salt

3 tbsp of Sweet Almond Oil

1 tbsp Ground oatmeal

6 Drops of Tea Tree oil

3 Drops of Petitgrain

3 Drops of Clary Sage

Dry Chest I

1/2 cup of Brown Sugar

3 tbsp of Sweet Almond Oil

1 tbsp Horsetail

3 Drops of Eucalyptus

4 Drops of Lavender

4 Drops of Geranium

2 Drops of Peppermint

Dry Chest II

1/2 cup of Brown Sugar

3 tbsp of Pure Aloe Juice

6 drops of Lavender

6 Drops of Chamomile

3 Drops of Patchouli

Normal Chest

1/2 cup of Brown Sugar

3 tbsp of Sweet Almond Oil

4 Drops Carrot Seed

4 Drops Petitgrain

4 Drops Ylang Ylang

Elbows and Knees-Regular

1/2 cup of Brown Sugar

3 tbsp of Sweet Almond Oil

4 Drops Ylang Tlang

4 Drops Lavender

4 Drops Rose

4 Drops Geranium

Elbows and Knees-scaly

We've all had those scaly, or hard skin almost like callouses, on our elbows and knees. You need to use a combination of herbs and essential oils that soften the skin and heating it will help to soften the hard skin on the joints.

1/2 Cup Brown Sugar

2 tbsp Pure Aloe Juice

1/2 tbsp Kelp

4 Drops Lavender

4 Drops Chamomile

2 Drops Petitgrain

- Gently heat to slightly above body temp.
- Apply while still warm

Elbows and Knees-dry

1/2 Cup Brown Sugar

2 tbsp Pure Aloe Juice

1/2 tbsp Kelp

4 Drops Carrot Oil

4 Drops Frankincense

Arms and Legs-Dry

1/2 cup Brown Sugar

3 tbsp Coconut oil

4 Drops Peppermint

4 Drops Clary Sage

4 Drops Rose

Arms and Legs-Rashes

There may be times when you have rash patches in the bends of your elbows and knees. Here are a couple of recipes for when that happens. This is for regular rashes, and not rashes that are raw, seeping, and in some cases, bleeding.

Recipe I

1/2 cup Brown Sugar

3 tbsp Coconut oil

4 Drops Patchouli

4 Drops Rose

4 Drops Geranium

Recipe II

1/2 cup Brown Sugar

3 tbsp Sweet Almond Oil

1/2 tbsp Tumeric

4 Drops Carrot Seed

4 Drops Frankincense

4 Drops Ylang Ylang

Cellulite Scrubs

Instead of putting a list of essential oils you can add to the list, I will simply say that citrus oils like grapefruit, Lime, and even lemon. They all stimulate blood flow and prevent lymph accumulation, and helps to tighten the skin.

Cellulite, the fat that makes your bottom and thighs look like cottage cheese, bumpy, lumpy, and unsightly. People spend thousands of dollars yearly to get rid of cellulite in order to look thinner. Some go to the gym and exercise it away, others pay for liposuction to get rid of it faster. Though exercise is an effective way to rid yourself of cellulite, you can give it a little boost with these scrubs.

Recipe I

1/2 cup Brown Sugar
3 tbsp Sweet Almond Oil
1/2 tbsp Kelp
8 Drops of Grapefruit
4 Drops Peppermint
4 Drops Chamomile

Recipe II

1/2 cup Brown Sugar
3 tbsp Sweet Almond Oil
1/2 tbsp Kelp
8 Drops of Lime oil
4 Drops Grapefruit
4 Drops Peppermint

Recipe III

1/2 cup Sea Salt

3 tbsp coconut oil

4 Drops Lemon

4 Drops Grapefruit

4 Drops Lavender

4 Drops Petitgrain

Chapter 4 - Callouses

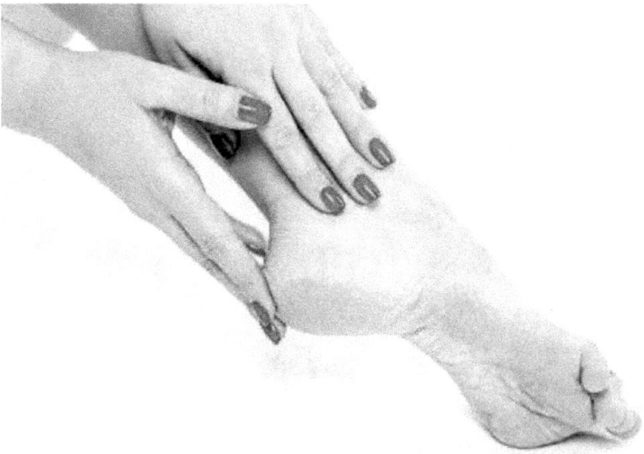

If you play instruments, craft, or even walk barefoot, you will develop a thick hard skin. This is called callouses. There are a few ways to get rid of the callouses.

Preventing Callouses

To prevent the formation of callouses on your feet, wear socks, shoes, or if you don't want to wear either, you can wear sandals or flip flops.

At the end of each day, soak your feet in warm water, pat them dry and apply moisturizer. After you've applied the moisturizer, put on socks to make sure the lotion stays on the feet.

It is a little trickier to prevent callouses on the fingers. You can place band aids on your finger before starting your craft work or practicing your string instruments. You can also buy picks that slip onto your fingers so your fingers do not touch the strings. There are also special tools for craft people you can fit onto the end of your fingers so you don't expose your finger tips to the wire or other materials.

Ingredients needed

Course Sea Salt

This is must for removing callouses. The salt has properties will help slough off the hard layers of the callouses to expose the new skin underneath.

Coconut Oil

This is the second ingredient that is valuable in removing callouses. It will help to soften the hard skin

For the Feet I

1/2 cup Course Sea Salt
3 tbsp Coconut oil
1 tbsp Orange Zest (the oils will help soften the callouses)
4 Drops Lemon
6 Drops Grapefruit
3 Drops Tea Tree oil
3 Drops Carrot Seed

For the Feet II

1/2 cup Course Sea Salt
3 tbsp Coconut oil
1 tbsp Ground Horsetail
4 Drops Lavender
4 Drops Chamomile
4 Drops Grapefruit

- gently warm the scrub
- Rub the callouses with the scrub until it cools
- Soak your feet in warm water with Epsom salts.

For the Hand and Fingers I

1/2 cup Medium Course Sea Salt

3 tbsp Coconut oil

1 tbsp ground Horsetail

6 Drops Lemon

6 Drops Rose

4 Drops Frankincense

For the Hand and Fingers II

1/2 cup Medium Course Sea Salt

3 tbsp Coconut oil

1 tbsp Kelp

6 Drops Lavender

4 Drops Lime

4 Drops Rose

Follow the directions for the feet to get the most out of the scrubs.

Chapter 5 - After the Scrub

Whether you've just cleared your rashes, blemishes or callouses, your maintenance doesn't stop there. You also need to stay on top of it to prevent having to use scrubs too often.

The Importance of Moisturizer

Using moisturizer can keep your skin from breaking out into acne and even maintaining elasticity of the skin to prevent your skin from breaking. Which type of moisturizer is good you?

Dry Skin

A moisturizer with aloe and lanolin can help with keeping your face smooth and supple.

To keep your body's skin smooth and moisturized, lotions like Gold Bond, Lubriderm, and even Intensive Care are all good options.

Oily Skin

You will need a light moisturizer for oily skin, and it should be applied after you have patted your face dry to lock in any moisture from washing it.
Light lotions are also good for the rest of your body as well.

Normal Skin

Regular moisturizers are easy to find and use when your skin is normal. Once a day, usually before bed, will keep your skin smooth, silky, and maintain your elasticity.

Callouses

Heavy moisturizers designed for the feet will provide the deep moisturizing your feet need to keep them soft and prevent the rebuilding of callouses on your feet. This should works on your hands as well.

Soaking your hands and feet will also help to soften the callouses to make it easy to remove. Just remember, you need to moisturize regularly to keep it from reforming.

Picking the right one

To pick the right moisturizer, you need one that absorbs into the skin quickly and doesn't leave your skin feeling greasy or oily. The problem with this is when you get into body butters. There is no non-greasy body butter you can use. These are best used before going to bed on the hands and feet. You can then cover your hands and feet with socks and gloves to make sure the butter gets absorbed into your skin for faster healing. It may take you a bit to find the right moisturizer.

Conclusion

Don't let this book be the only book you ever own now that you have started your journey to learning about natural health. Look online for more resources on herbs, essential oils, and even herbal extracts and teas. You can join online groups and forums to help further your new interest and gain more knowledge on natural health.

If you are looking for recommendations on books to get you started, here is a short list:
-Today's Herbal Health, Lousie Tenney
-The Illustrated Encyclopedia of Essential Oils, Julia Lawless

There are also websites to get you started on your journey further into essential oils:
aromaweb.com
moutainroseherbs.com

Stay away from sites like DoTerra which can give you bad advice on the usage of essential oils. Stick with sites that have been up for 10 years or more.

When shopping for essential oils, do your homework. Find out how long the company has been around, how they test for purity, and make sure what you are buying is the pure essential oil. There are companies out there that will try to pass diluted oils as pure or a different essential oil than the one stated. There are essential oils that have similar names. It is for this reason I included the Latin name of the essential oil. Each oil acts differently on the skin.

Do a patch test before you start using the essential oil to see if you have a reaction. Add three drops of an essential oil to one teaspoon of any type of carrier oil and mix well. Then choose a small patch of skin to rub it in. Wait overnight. If you do not have any type of discoloration or rash, your are good. Any type of discoloration and you need to find and use another oil.
I hope this book provided you with the information you needed to get you started. Until next time, be well.

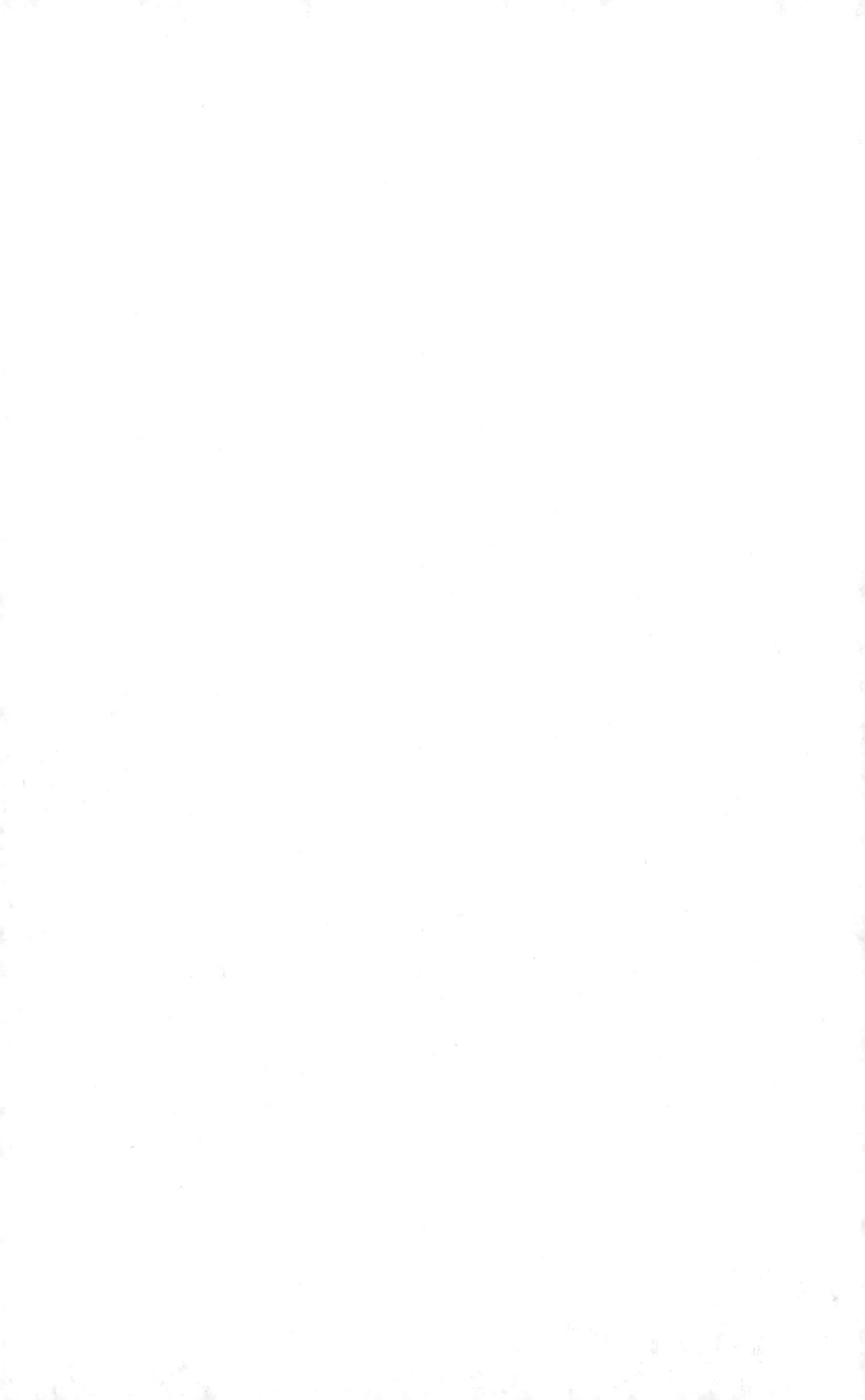